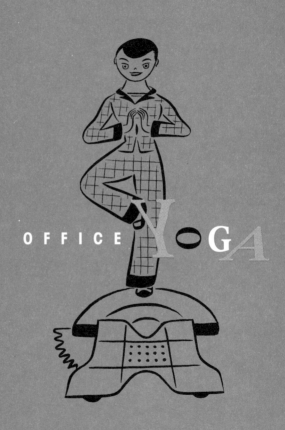

OFFICE Y·O·G·A

OFFICE YOGA

Simple Stretches for Busy People

BY Darrin Zeer

ILLUSTRATIONS BY Michael Klein

CHRONICLE BOOKS

SAN FRANCISCO

Library of Congress Cataloging-in-Publication Data available.

ISBN 0-8118-2685-6

Printed in Singapore

Designed by Brett MacFadden

Distributed in Canada by Raincoast Books
9050 Shaughnessy Street
Vancouver, British Columbia V6P 6E5

10 9 8 7 6

Chronicle Books LLC
85 Second Street
San Francisco, California 94105

www.chroniclebooks.com

THIS BOOK IS DEDICATED TO ALL OF YOU.

May it inspire you to

take good care of yourself

at the office and throughout the day.

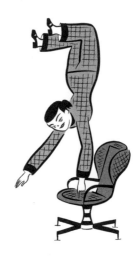

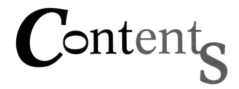

Contents

Quick Help *Guide*

Introduction

You're stuck in another marathon meeting. Your back and neck are screaming; your brain is swimming. You come home stressed and exhausted, wanting nothing more than a pizza and a video before going to sleep to get up and do it all over again tomorrow.

How can you get relief?

Let's face it: If exercise isn't simple and easy, most of us won't do it. If we can't fit it comfortably into our daily routine, we'll never stick with it.

Try a few of the yoga stretches in this book. They are designed so they can be done anywhere, anytime, whether you're in your office, in meetings, on the phone, or even in bed. These stretches are gentle and relaxing; they will soothe aching muscles; they will ease your tension whether you have a spare twenty minutes during lunch or only two between phone calls.

The philosophy and practice of yoga comes from India. *Yoga* basically means union, bringing together the physical, emotional, and spiritual parts of ourselves. Yoga is not only about the well-being of our bodies; it is a path toward deeper meaning in life.

In the ancient Sanskrit language, yoga stretches or postures are called *asanas,* which means to sit or dwell quietly in a particular position. Asanas are said to bring steadiness, stability, ease, and happiness to one's life.

Yoga asanas help you on many levels: They will strengthen you physically, assisting the digestive, immune, and other bodily systems, and they will empower your mind to be calm, alert, and focused. Once you begin to do them with ease throughout the day, you'll be surprised how powerful these simple stretches really are.

This book integrates this age-old wisdom into the modern workplace. Yoga stretching is a natural fit in any office, becoming an oasis of calm in a hectic day, one that maintains your physical health and restores your vibrant alertness.

Give it a chance to work for you. Go ahead and open to a page; imitate the figure, ease into the stretch, read an inspirational quote. Enjoy the good feeling. If you have a few nagging problems, turn to the Quick Help Guide on page 7.

Thanks for trying.

Five Essential Tips for Breathing and Stretching

1. Most important: When stretching, do not hold your breath. Breathe deeply and slowly, in rhythm with your movements.

2. While stretching, focus on relaxing your entire body. Pay attention to the areas that remain tense.

3. If you want to go deeper into a stretch, breathe and relax into it. Don't force it.

4. If a stretch hurts, don't do it. In other words: "If pain, no gain."

5. In a hurry? Do one or two stretches fully rather than rushing through many.

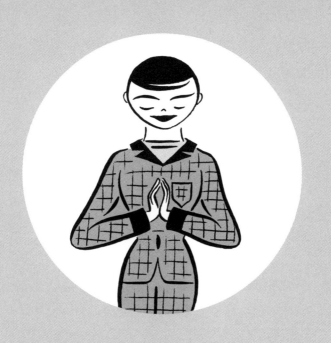

morning eye

Openers

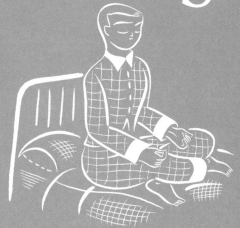

Rise and *Shine*

First thing in the morning, practice this two-minute calming meditation.

> Sit up in bed and breathe gently into your belly.
>
> Feel your body soften and your mind relax.
>
> Focus on the day's activities.
>
> Think about what you want to accomplish and what the day will bring.
>
> Breathe deeply.

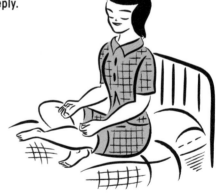

"The quieter you become, the more you are able to hear."

–Baba Ram Dass

Yoga in *Bed*

Wake up with these gentle stretches. Remember to do them slowly, breathe deeply, and relax.

Lie on your back in bed.

Bring both knees to your chest and wrap your arms around them.

Breathe deeply and feel your lower back release.

Drop both knees to one side, keeping your shoulders flat; relax in the stretch.

Gently bring both legs back up, and switch sides.

Knees at your chest again, rock back and forth.

If you can, raise up into a forward bend, chest out, upper body stretching forward.

Take hold of your legs.

Relax your shoulders and drop your head.

Take several deep full-body breaths, stretching a little farther each time. Don't push it.

To go deeper into the stretch, wrap a belt or towel around your feet, hold both ends, and gently stretch forward.

Gentle Sun Salutations

This gentle series of yoga postures helps wake up the entire body. Take the first round slow and easy; if you become dizzy, lie flat on your back and rest. As you become more adept at the postures, your breath should fall into a rhythm like the waves of the ocean.

First, place your hands in a prayer position and inhale deeply. Reach your hands up high and stretch, arching slightly back. Exhaling, sweep your outstretching arms forward and down till you are bent over, touching the floor if you can; relax your head and neck and take a few breaths. Squat down, place your hands flat on the ground, take a big step back with your left foot, and stretch, arching up with your back. Step back with your right foot and rest both knees on the ground, making a table with your body; first stretch your head up and curve your lower back down, then drop your head down and arch your back up. Repeat once and breathe in rhythm as you do.

With your hands and the soles of your feet on the ground, lift your buttocks toward the sky, keeping your arms and legs straight and your heels down; stay as long as comfortable. Drop down onto your hands and knees,

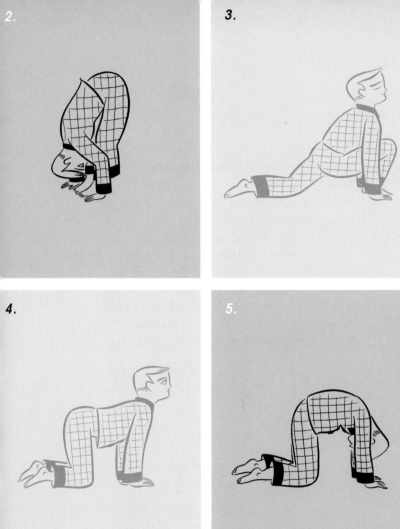

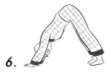

6.

sit on your calves, and lower your upper body to the ground with your arms outstretched on the floor. Relax for a few breaths. Raise back up on your hands and knees and bring your left foot forward, so it's underneath you, with your right leg stretched back. Arch your back upward and breathe. Bring your right foot forward, straighten your legs with your upper body hanging down, and slowly walk your hands up your legs into a standing position. Raise your arms toward the sky and stretch back slightly, tightening your buttocks. Exhale as you return your hands to the beginning prayer position, then relax.

Rest for a few moments, breathing deeply and rhythmically, then repeat as many times as you want or as time permits.

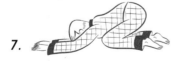

7.

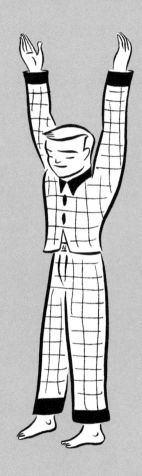

Relaxation on the Run

If you jog in the morning (or anytime), remember to relax as you exercise. Keep your back straight and your arms and shoulders loose. Shake out your hands and feel your chest stretching out as you breathe deeply.

"Everything has beauty, but not everyone sees it."

—Confucius

Power Breakfast *Smoothie*

Feed your body and your mind–it only takes a minute.
Mix together in a blender:

> soy or regular milk
>
> real juice
>
> frozen berries
>
> a banana
>
> soy or whey protein powder
>
> whatever else you desire—be creative.

Pour into a travel cup and go!

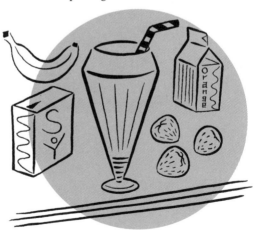

Red Light Rejuvenation

This also works on planes and trains.

Sit back, relax, and gently roll your head in circles.

Shrug your shoulders up and down, breathing in rhythm as you do.

Become one with the traffic flow.

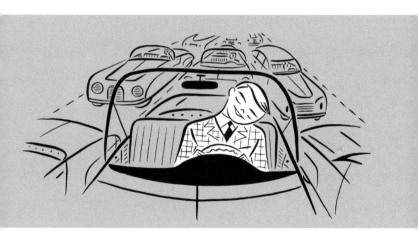

Antidote for Road Rage

Stop-and-go traffic making you nuts? Loosen up your
windpipes and sing your favorite song. Imitate an
opera singer and come from your belly with the sound.

"Better late than never."

—Titus Livius

at-the-desk

Relaxation

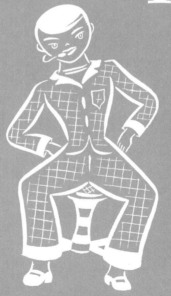

Office Yoga Posture

Want to ease your back pain and improve and energize
your mood at the same time? Good posture is the best
start. Throughout the day and when preparing for your
Office Yoga stretches, take a moment to align your
body properly.

Most important is to sit on your sit bones; to
find these sharp bones, place your hands under
your buttocks and rock forward and back.

Notice how, when you rise forward, your body
aligns on top of your sit bones; immediately
your back straightens, your chest expands, and
your shoulders, neck, and head rise and align.

Now sit back on your tailbone—everything
slumps and drops, including your mood!

Rise forward again. Feel your spine lift into a
straight line all the way up to your head.

Let your shoulders relax, soften your jaw, lower
your chin, and take a few deep calm breaths.

Can you feel the difference? This simple shift in posture improves not only your physical well-being but
your confidence and sense of self.

Keyboard Calisthenics

Do stretches with your hands and wrists as often as possible. Improvise–be creative!

> **With hands in a prayer position, move in all directions and stretch.**
>
> **Squeeze fists tight.**
>
> **Stretch fingers wide.**
>
> **Interlace fingers and rotate hands.**
>
> **Invent stretches that feel good.**

Make it a habit: Constantly stretch your hands and wrists.

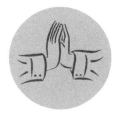 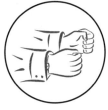 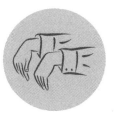

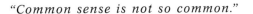

"Common sense is not so common."

–Voltaire

Neck Rolls

Drop your head to one side.

Roll it around in a wide circle; switch directions.

Slowly find the tight spots.

Hold and breathe, letting your breath release the tightness.

Extra stretch: Place a hand on your head and gently pull to the side.

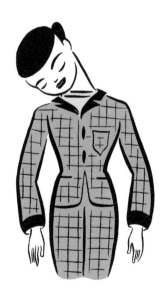

Arm Pulls

Place left arm behind your back.

Grab your wrist with your right hand.

Drop your head to the right side.

Roll head slightly and explore any tightness.

Stretch and breathe.

Repeat with other arm.

Bend left arm above and behind your head.

Grab your elbow with your right hand and stretch up.

Breathe and let shoulders relax.

Repeat with other arm.

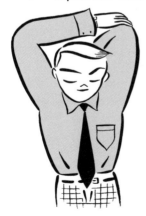

Kick Back Log-on Pose

Interlace your fingers behind your head.

Relax your elbows and shoulders.

Smile, breathe, and stretch your elbows back.

Let the tightness release slowly.

Repeat throughout the day.

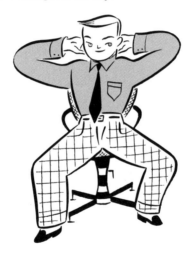

"Let the beauty of what you love be what you do."

—Rumi

Human Basketball Net

Raise your arms straight above your head.

Interlace your fingers.

Alternate palms downward and upward.

Stretch and breathe.

Stretch your arms out in front and relax your shoulders.

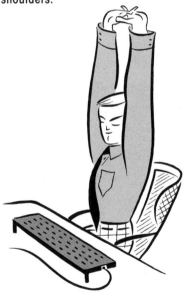

Reaching Hands

First Stretch:

> Hold your arms out to the side.
>
> Stretch with your fingertips to the opposite walls.
>
> Breathe and relax.

Second Stretch:

> Arms outstretched, shoulders relaxed, palms down.
>
> Tilt hands upward and stretch forearms.
>
> Hold as long as comfortable.
>
> Stretch hands down, breathe, and hold.

Third Stretch:

> Arms outstretched.
>
> Slowly tilt sideways like a windmill.
>
> Reach for the floor and ceiling.
>
> Gently stretch the mid-area.

"Learning is movement from moment to moment."

—Krishnamurti

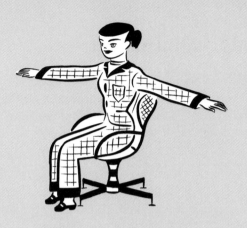

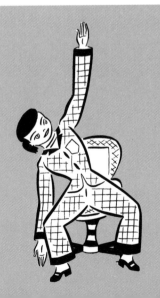

E-mail Meditation

While you are reading your e-mail, remember to breathe slowly and focus your attention on your breath. Make the out-breath two times longer than the in-breath. This will immediately calm you.

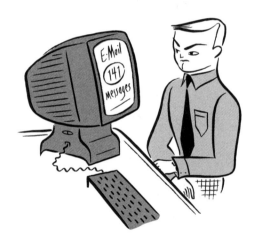

"Kind words can be short and easy to speak, but their echoes are truly endless."

—Mother Teresa

Open Chest Stretch

Sit near the edge of the chair.

Hold the sides of the seat.

Gently stretch up and forward.

Open your chest and tilt your head back.

Relax and breathe into the stretch.

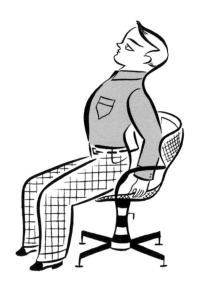

What to Watch Out For

Over 60 percent of all workplace ailments are repetitive strain injuries. They can be healed with early diagnosis. If you have constant pain in the hands, wrists, or forearms, see a physician for assistance.

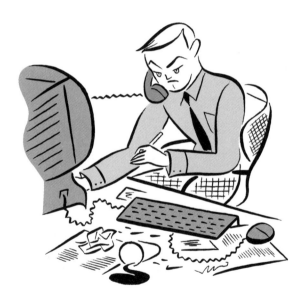

Feeling Good!

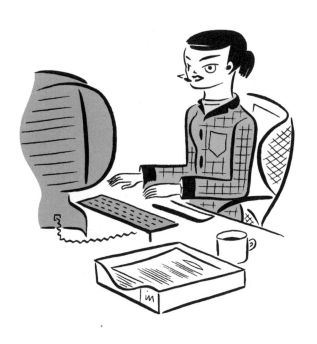

Circling Torso

Sit forward with your feet flat on the ground, hands on hips (if you can), and relax your shoulders. Begin to rotate your torso in circles. Explore with your whole body, relax, and breathe.

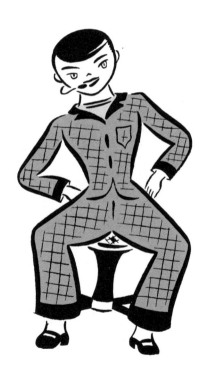

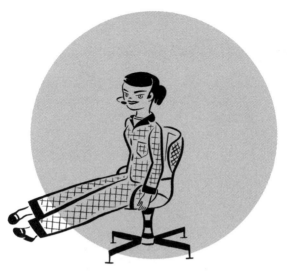

Feet and Ankles

While you talk on the phone, stretch your legs out and
rotate your ankles and feet. Notice your attention
increase as you stretch.

Headache Solution

Place your index fingers in the middle and just above each eyebrow, press with your fingers, and hold. Close eyes and breathe deeply.

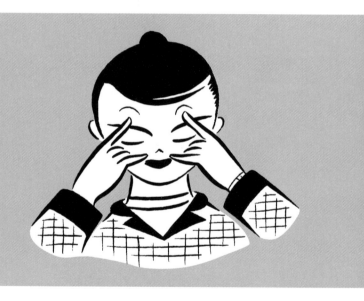

Eye Strain *Solution*

Take minibreaks from your computer screen as you work.

> Refocus every ten minutes by looking out the window or around the office.
>
> Each hour close your eyes, let your face soften.
>
> Slowly roll eyes in a circle.
>
> Take a few breaths, and return to action.

For soothing relief, rub palms together very fast till they get warm, then place them gently over your eyes. Softly hold them there till the heat dissipates.

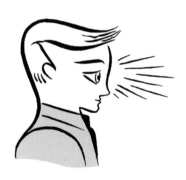

Natural Face Lift

It really works!

Pretend to chew a large piece of gum up and down and side to side, mouth open.

Squeeze your eyes shut and lift your eyebrows up and down.

Massage your cheekbones, forehead, and temples with your fingers and knuckles.

Knead your brows with your fingertips.

Make sure shoulders are relaxed.

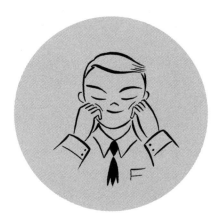

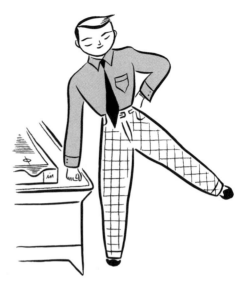

Leg Kicks

Stand in front of your desk with an open space behind you.

Steady yourself with both hands and kick your leg back with the knee slightly bent.

Stretch and take a deep breath and slowly drop leg to the ground.

Repeat and switch sides.

Turn to the side and stretch leg out.

Relax your body and keep standing leg strong, body straight.

Switch sides.

Balance Tree Pose

Try this just before a big meeting or call.

Remove shoes and stand next to a table or chair for balance.

Raise right foot up against the inside of thigh.

Place right hand on foot if it slides down.

If you feel steady, place hands by chest in prayer position.

Feel the standing foot rooted into the ground.

Relax and breathe.

Stand straight and balanced.

Switch legs slowly.

"Do it big, do it right, and do it with style."

—Fred Astaire

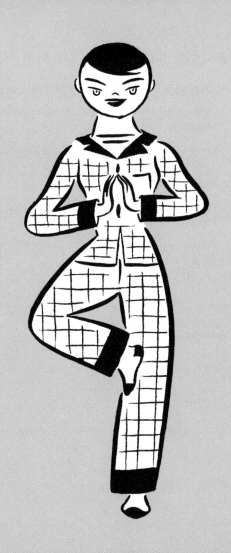

Close the Deal Warrior Pose

Raise your arms to the side with fingers pointed.

Take a big step to the side, with your right foot turned out and knee bent.

Keep your left foot planted, your leg straight.

Your upper body should be straight and strong, shoulders relaxed.

Don't hold your breath! Relax into the stretch and then gently release.

Return to a standing position, switch sides, and repeat.

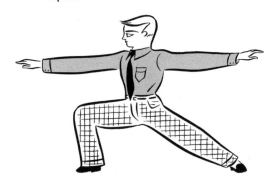

"Make haste slowly."

—Zen master

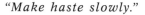

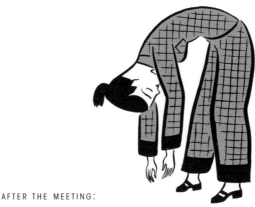

Ragdoll Pose

Let it all out with this re-energizing stretch.

> Take a deep breath.
>
> Arms straight up and stretch.
>
> Exhale, bend knees, and drop hands to ground.
>
> Relax your head and shoulders and take deep full-body breaths.
>
> Let everything sag toward the ground while still bent over.
>
> Return to standing position by slowly walking hands up legs.

Morning Meltdown *Stretch*

Find a quiet spot for this one.

> Lean facedown over a table.
>
> Keep feet on or near the ground.
>
> Comfortably breathe and relax.
>
> Feel your whole body weight resting on the table.
>
> Be gentle with your lower back.
>
> A towel or pillow feels good under your midsection.
>
> Take your time and relax into the stretch.

"It is not the answer that enlightens, but the question."

—Eugene Ionesco

To Do Today

Maintain a current to-do list by the day, week, month, and future.

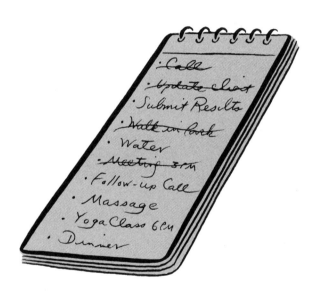

Where Did I Put that *Disk?*

Mess can equal stress.

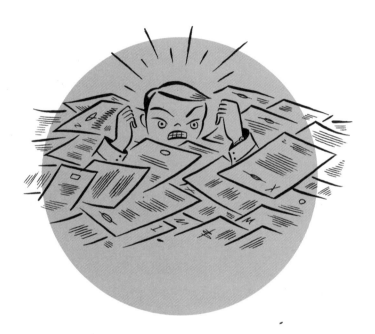

Clean It Out

Clean out the desk, hard drive, briefcase, car, everything.

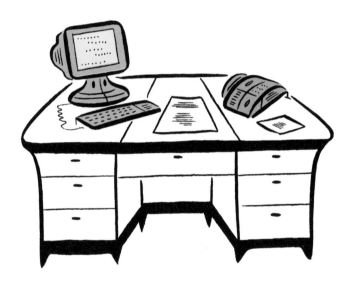

Stress Breaks!

Put this on your calendar! Schedule times in your week to relax and rejuvenate. Maybe just a five-minute stretch break after each meeting. Or better yet, treat yourself and your body to a lunchtime massage, hot bath, Jacuzzi, or walk around the block.

Remember, you will work better and smarter if you do.

"You're only as young as the last time you changed your mind."

—Timothy Leary

Self-Massage

Try these anytime.

Place both hands on your shoulders and neck.

Squeeze with your fingers and palms.

Rub vigorously.

Keep shoulders relaxed.

Wrap one hand around the other forearm.

Squeeze the muscles with thumb and fingers.

Move up and down from your elbow to fingertips and back again.

Repeat with other arm.

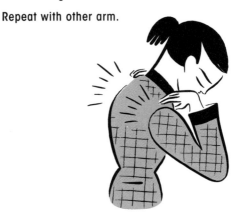

lunchtime

Escapes

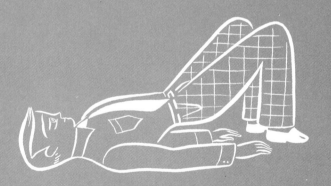

The World's Easiest *Diet*

You'll feel better if you eat well.

> Snack on fruit or nuts whenever you're hungry.
>
> Order a salad with your meal.
>
> Once in a while, eat light.
>
> Skip the quick fixes like sugar and caffeine.
>
> Drink herbal tea.

Most important of all: Use your lunch like a meditation. No calls or typing while you eat.

Drink!

Whenever you feel tired, drink lots of water. Fatigue is a common symptom of dehydration.

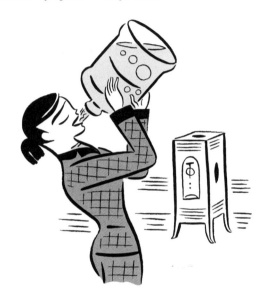

"Your work is to discover your work, and then with all your heart to give yourself to it."

–Buddha

Cobra Pose

Change into sweats at lunch and keep your back
healthy with this series of stretches.

Beginner's Cobra

Lie on your stomach, your forearms on the
ground.

Keep your elbows beneath your shoulders,
slightly supporting your raised upper body.

Keep your hips on the ground and your buttocks
tight to support your lower back.

Gently lift your head and chest.

Breathe and stretch, letting the tight areas
release.

Hold and breathe.

When ready, gently lower yourself to the ground.
Repeat.

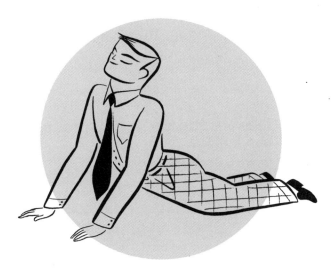

Full Cobra

Practice this stretch if the Beginner's Cobra is easy, but skip if you have lower back problems.

> Lie on stomach, hands under shoulders, palms down, elbows in.
>
> Lift your head and chest by slowly contracting your lower back muscles.
>
> Use your arm strength for support.
>
> Breathe deeply and relax.

Cat Pose

Get on your hands and knees to begin each Cat Pose.

Cat Cow

Raise your head up and arch your lower back down.

Exhale as you drop your head and arch your lower back up.

Move slowly, stretch deeply.

Repeat.

Cat Stretch

Gently lower your body onto your calves with your arms stretched out.

Relax your head and neck.

Breathe and rest. Feel your lower back release.

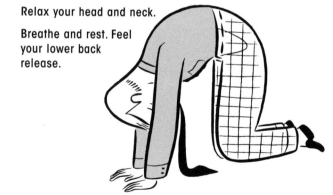

Belly and *Hips*

Lie on your back to begin each of the following
Healthy Back Stretches.

Half Sit-Ups

> Bend legs and cross arms over chest.
>
> Breathe deep and slowly sit halfway up.
>
> Pause. Feel your belly tighten.
>
> Breathe, release, rest, and repeat.

Hip Raises

> Bend legs, arms at your side and palms down.
>
> Gently raise your hips and hold.
>
> Breathe, release, and repeat.

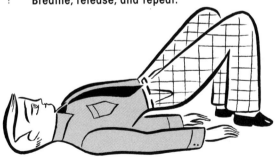

Full-Body Twist

Knee to Chest

Interlace fingers around your right knee.

Stretch your knee toward your chest, hips on the floor.

Breathe and hold.

Release, then switch legs.

Knee Over Leg

Pull right knee to your chest.

Take a deep breath and gently bend your right knee over your left leg.

Hold your right knee down with your left hand over the knee.

Turn your head in the opposite direction.

Take deep gentle breaths and relax your whole body. Keep both shoulders down.

Gently release, then switch legs.

"To know that you do not know is the best."

—Lao-tzu

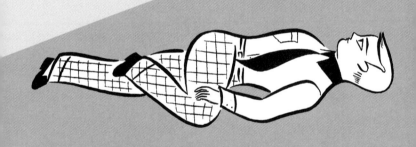

Knees Up

Sometimes the most powerful stretches are the easiest ones.

> Interlace fingers or arms around bent knees.
>
> Gently stretch your knees to chest, keeping your hips on the floor.
>
> Hold the stretch. Breathe into your lower back.
>
> Relax your body, and rest in the pose.

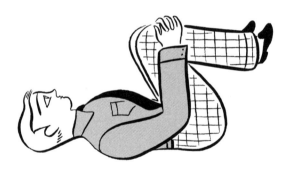

"Work is love made visible."

–Kahlil Gibran

Child's Posture

This is a gentle, relaxing stretch for your lower back.

Sit on calves and lay upper body on legs.

Place arms at your side.

Turn face to one side or lay forehead on ground.

Let your body relax and breathe.

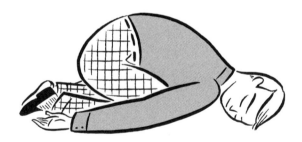

afternoon

Invigoration

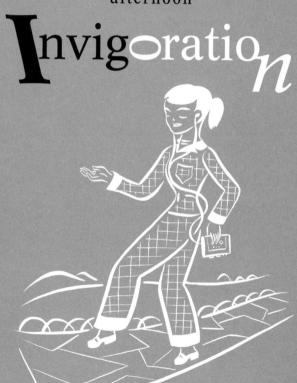

Crowded Elevator *Stretch*

Place hand on a wall for balance.

Standing on your left foot, cross right foot over left leg just above the ground.

Feel the sole of your left foot rooted into the floor, lengthen your body.

Relax and breathe, then switch legs.

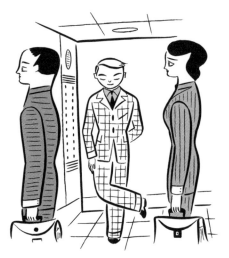

"To be uncertain is uncomfortable, but to be certain is ridiculous."

—Chinese proverb

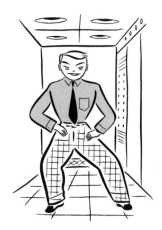

Empty Elevator *Stretches*

Place your right hand on a wall.

Stand up straight and bend your left leg back.

With your left hand, hold your toes and pull your foot to your buttocks.

Breathe, hold, release, and switch sides.

Place your hands on your hips.

With your legs apart, bend both knees slightly.

Make wide circles with your hips.

Reverse directions and breathe.

Photocopier Stretch

Place your hands on the edge of the copier.

Stand back with feet apart.

Drop your head and chest.

Breathe and relax your shoulders.

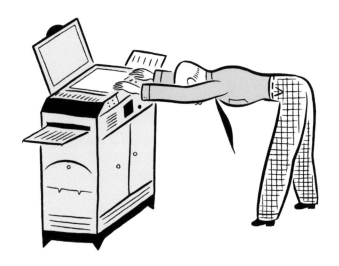

Late Client *Stretch*

Place both hands on the doorjambs at shoulder height, feet hip-width apart.

Gently let your body stretch forward.

Relax your head and breathe.

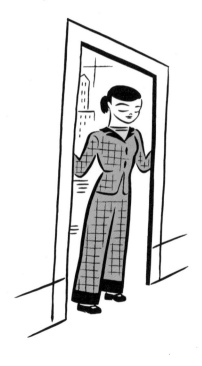

Practice Loving *Kindness*

Deliver a surprise decaf, low-fat latte to your cube mate.

Surprise someone with flowers . . .

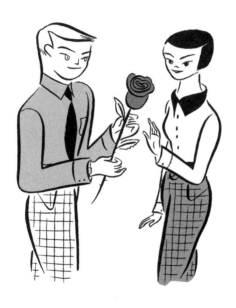

"No one's head aches when he is comforting another."

—Indian proverb

Allow yourself to do nothing *and be* completely bored!

Do this like a meditation.

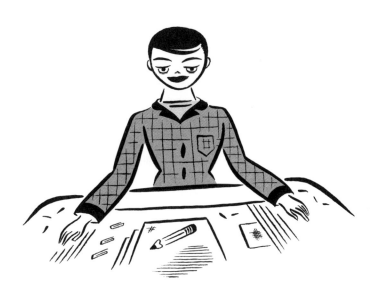

"Live to learn and you will learn to live."
—Portuguese proverb

Focus on This Moment

Here's a good way to focus when your mind gets distracted.

Alternate Nostril Breathing

> Using your right hand, place your thumb against your right nostril.
>
> Inhale deeply through your left nostril.
>
> Hold your breath and close your left nostril with your index finger.
>
> Release your right thumb and exhale slowly through your right nostril.
>
> Repeat, inhaling on the right and exhaling on the left.
>
> Let each breath become longer. Feel the calm and balance.

Keep It Simple

Take one step at a time, breathe, and be calm.

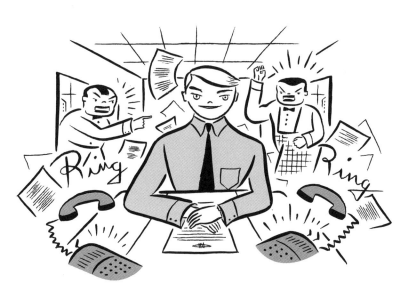

"Patience is the companion of wisdom."

−St. Augustine

Energize Anytime

Shake your hands and arms.

Shake each leg and foot, one at a time.

Swing your arms in wide circles—up and around and from side to side.

Switch directions.

Wiggle your whole body till it feels loose.

Raise both arms above your head.

Take left wrist with your right hand and gently stretch to the right.

Breathe into the stretch.

Keep your body straight and strong.

Switch sides and repeat.

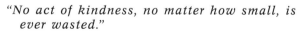

"No act of kindness, no matter how small, is ever wasted."

– Aesop

Hands Behind *Back*

Interlace your fingers behind your back.

Gently bend forward.

Stretch your hands and arms up and back.

Breathe into the stretch.

Gently release arms.

With fists, tap lower back and legs.

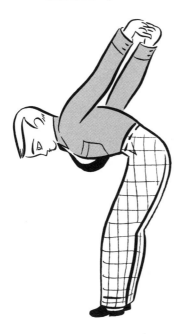

On-the-Run *Stretch*

Lift your right foot onto a solid desk or table.

Turn your standing foot to the side for balance.

Stretch over your leg, placing your hands on your leg or on the table.

Relax your head. Breathe into the stretch.

Flex your foot, breathe.

Relax your foot, breathe.

Switch legs and repeat.

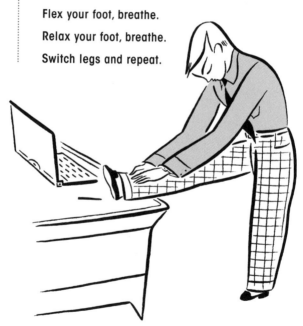

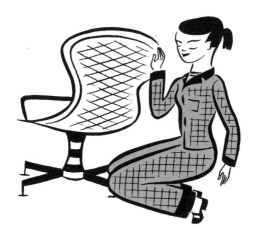

Power Leg Bends

Place your hand on a solid chair to steady yourself.

Keeping your back straight, bend your knees, lower body slowly, and then raise up.

Do this several times slowly, breathing in rhythm.

Try this with your feet down or heels up.

"The moment we want to be something we are no longer free."

–Krishnamurti

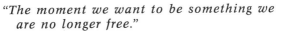

Oh My God I'm Never Going to Make It

Take a break, go for a walk, visualize your in-box as fan mail.

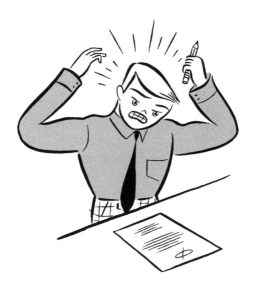

"*The road up and the road down is one and the same.*"

—Heraclitus

Afternoon Meltdown

Back sore? Legs tired? Mind racing?

Find a quiet spot near a chair or wall.

Lay on your back and put your legs up.

Breathe.

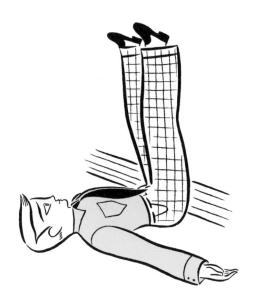

Afternoon Power Walk

Relax and renew.

> Head outside.
>
> Walk vigorously for ten minutes.
>
> Focus on breathing.
>
> Observe the people and nature around you.

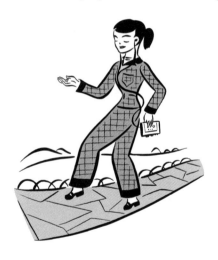

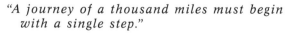

"A journey of a thousand miles must begin with a single step."

—Lao-tzu

Hang In There Stretches

Chair Boogie

Interlace fingers below your knee.

Bend leg up.

Stretch forehead to knee.

Switch legs.

Spinal Twist

While sitting, cross your left leg over your right.

Place your right hand or elbow on the crossed knee.

Gently turn your body to the left and look behind you.

Switch legs and twist the other way.

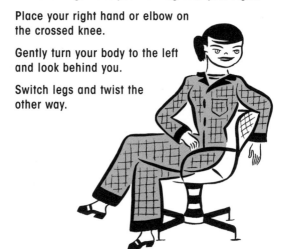

Let It Go, Let It Out

When you're done for the day, release all your tension.

> While sitting, reach your hands toward the sky.
>
> Breathe in deeply and relax completely on the exhale.
>
> Drop your arms and upper body toward the ground like a rag doll.

Make sure you're alone before trying this Lion Pose!

> While at your desk, take a deep breath and roar as loud as you can. Come from your belly with the sound, and open your mouth as wide as you can.

"He who knows others is wise;
He who knows himself is enlightened."

—Lao-tzu

Breathing Meditation

Place one hand on your belly.

Breathe slow and deep.

Feel your hand rise and fall.

Let your shoulders drop.

Feel your body relax and renew.

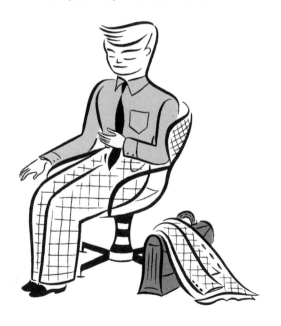

evening

Balancers

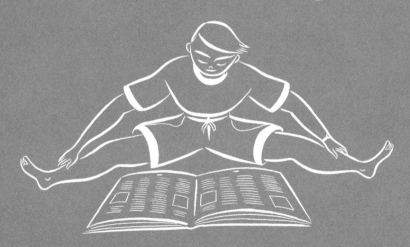

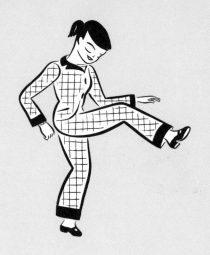

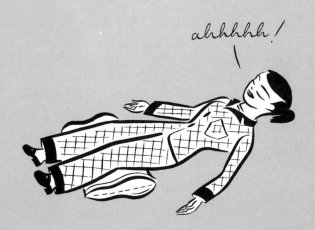

ahhhhh!

Getting Home *Release*

Twist and Shout

> Put on your favorite music, and for two to five
> minutes, simply let your hair down. Free-flow
> dance and stretch. Focus on letting go of your
> day and relaxing.

Rest and Relax

> For two to five minutes, lie down on your back
> and let your thoughts go. Get comfortable, per-
> haps placing a pillow under your knees. Take
> easy breaths. Imagine your body sinking into the
> ground. Relax the tight spots, calm the mind,
> feel peace.

Yoga for Couch *Potatoes*

While Watching TV

> Sit on floor.
>
> Bend your legs and bring the soles of your feet together, close to your body.
>
> Grab your feet with your hands, and gently lower your knees.
>
> Raise your chest and breathe.

While Reading the Paper

> Sit on floor.
>
> Stretch your legs out straight and wide apart.
>
> Slowly walk your hands down your legs.
>
> Gently raise chest up.
>
> Take a few breaths, then drop your head and shoulders down.
>
> Breathe and relax.

"Cherish that which is within you."

—Chuang-tzu

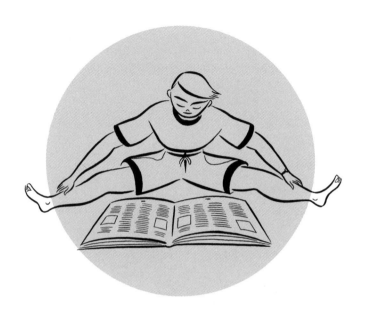

Take a Bath

To relax and renew, treat yourself to a mini-spa night.
Run a hot tub, put on some soft music, light candles.
Use bath oils and salts.

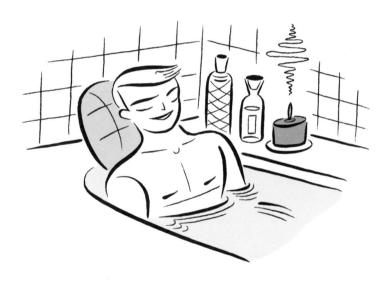

"It takes a long time to become young."

– Pablo Picasso

Get a Good Night's *Sleep*

Can't sleep? Drink some herbal tea. Do a calming
meditation. Play some soft music or nature sounds.

"The journey is the reward."

—Tao saying

Acknowledgments

Louis and Carole Zeer
John Mapleback
My editor, Sarah Malarkey
Associate Editor, Mikyla Bruder
Monique Jaspers

The Lady, David Swanson, Kalindi La Gourasana, Rob Zeer, Cynthia Ehman, Michelle Courage, Nita Abraham, Stan Ravinsky, Cynthia Zeito, and everyone at Chronicle Books.

My friends around the globe: Mazzarati, Cheri, Scott, Abheeru, Xian, Troy, Karen, Mary-Ann, Arynne and Bill Simon, Carl, Cassio, Takako, Dave, Mike, Carol, Peri, Dean, Sammi, Earl, Alejandro, Eldert, Sean and Shawn, Sumi, Stephen, Ryan, Allan, Sally, Linda, Beth, Owen, Bill and "Big" John, Fann, Gisela, and the many others. I couldn't have done it without all of you; thank you for your support.

Biographies

DARRIN ZEER has been practicing and teaching yoga for more than twelve years. He spent seven years in Asia, traveling and studying many of the Eastern arts of healing, meditation, and physical therapies as well as different forms of yoga.

Darrin has staffed the Miracle of Love intensive for the last six years. This intensive is a nine-day transformational workshop that attracts some eighty participants from around the world every month.

He is currently in private practice with individuals and groups in the Los Angeles and San Diego areas. His focus is on coaching people to have more peace and joy in their bodies and lives as well as teaching simple tools to relieve stress at work and at home.

If you or your company would like to make contact, check out **www.relaxyoga.com.**

MICHAEL KLEIN is an award-winning illustrator who lives just outside of New York City. His illustrations have appeared in a wide range of publications including the *New York Times, Newsweek, Forbes,* and *Natural Health.* His work was also featured in *The Working Stiff Cookbook,* published by Chronicle Books.

The Ultimate *State*

OFFICE NIRVANA

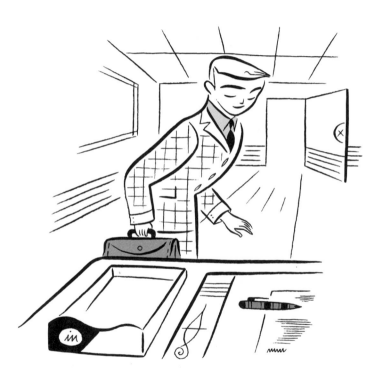